ENJOY ROUND-THE-CLOCK SUPPORT – ONLINE!

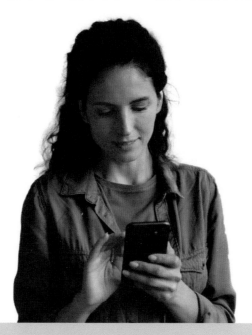

SCOTTISH SLIMMERS DIGITAL TRACKER

Download the mobile and web app FREE

Our comprehensive online service gives you the tools to:

- Track what you eat in your personal Daily Journal
- Browse and add Check counted Scottish Slimmers recipes
- Search 500 brands for Check-counted foods
- Track your weight loss progress

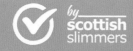

Redcurrants
Strawberries
Clementines
Grapefruit
Raspberries
Mandarins
Passion
Apricots
Blackberries
Berries
Lemon
Satsumas
Gooseberries
fruit
Lime
Melon
Nectarine
Tangerines
Cherries
Plums
PearOrange
Blackcurrants
Rhubarb
Peach
Pomegranate
Cranberries
Blueberries
Apple

Published by Scottish Slimmers Limited

ISBN 978-1-904462-02-6

For more information about Scottish Slimmers visit

www.scottishslimmers.com

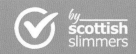

TABLE OF CONTENTS

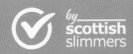

WELCOME TO SCOTTISH SLIMMERS

If you're reading this, it's because you have decided you are ready to lose weight. Maybe your health has become a priority, or you want freedom from fretting about what you eat, or you recognise that dropping a dress size (or more) will help you feel better about yourself. Whatever your motivation, Scottish Slimmers is here to help.

Joining Scottish Slimmers is not about a diet, it's about developing a healthier relationship with food, and we are by your side, keeping you on track all the way to your Target Weight – and beyond.

Scottish Slimmers' unique Checks system is designed for flexibility and has been effective for thousands of people, just like you, for more than 40 years.

At Scottish Slimmers, we believe in enjoying food! We believe in small, simple food and lifestyle changes for a healthy, sustainable weight loss. We focus on how you feel, your well-being and your motivation, not just your weight on the scales.

Our flexible approach lets you choose how you lose, following the plan that suits your life then doing it your own way; create your own menus or select from thousands of Scottish Slimmers recipes, but always eating the food you love.

Simply by staying within your daily Check allowance, you will get great weight losses every week. And with Everyday Essentials (EE) your body gets its daily nutritional boost keeping you feeling satisfied inside and out... because it all starts with YOU!

BE PREPARED
Recognise your weaknesses – we all have them! – and plan how to avoid or overcome them.

BELIEVE IN YOURSELF
Have the confidence to believe you can and think of past failures stepping stones to success.

LEARN FORGIVENESS
When things don't go to plan, remember every day is a new opportunity to start fresh.

CELEBRATE SUCCESS
Every positive step towards your Target Weight will do wonders to boost your confidence.

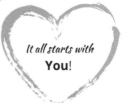

It all starts with **You**!

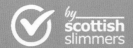

CHOOSE HOW YOU LOSE

With Scottish Slimmers, you can choose how you lose! Each plan encourages you to eat tasty, filling food that's good for you – and you can swap between plans whenever you want.

Our Eating Plans are designed to make lifestyle changes easy - packed with family-friendly food, for recipes and menus that put you back in control.

... the freedom & flexibility of FeelGood Food or keep count with Classic Checks... you choose!

FEELGOOD FOOD PLAN:

You eat healthy, filling foods from the FeelGood Food lists. As long as you choose food from the FeelGood categories, you don't have to count Checks or measure*.

You do have to count Checks for any food or drinks not in the FeelGood categories. You have weekly allowance of FlexiChecks for these.

CLASSIC CHECKS:

Every food and drink has a Check value, and you have a daily Check allowance PLUS a weekly FlexiChecks allowance. You can eat and drink anything you like, simply count your Checks and stay within your allowance to lose. This plan gives you maximum flexibility to eat the food you like, when you like.

PLUS EVERYDAY ESSENTIALS

Some foods are essential for your health and more important to ensure balanced, nutritious eating habits. We label these **Everyday Essentials,** and these are logged separately in the App and a bonus on top of your allowances.

*recommended adult portions equivalent

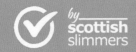

FIND THE PLAN THAT WORKS FOR YOU

Scottish Slimmers understands that life doesn't revolve around food but making decisions about what you eat and when can be the difference between success or failure.

Most people eat about the same amount over a week, although usually a little less on some days and a little more on others.

If you're not sure which of our Eating Plans will work for you, consider your personality and lifestyle before choosing which Plan to follow.

Weight loss is easy when it fits your lifestyle...

How would you describe yourself – A or B?

	A	B
I'm generally...	Organised	Disorganised
My schedule is...	Relaxed	Structured
I love...	Home Cooked	Eating Out
I prefer...	Meals Times	Grazing
My lunch is...	Packed Lunch	Bought Lunch
I prefer...	All you can eat	Measured Serving

IF YOU WERE MOSTLY A, TRY FOLLOWING FEELGOOD FOOD:

Eat healthy, nutritious food from the Feelgood lists. As long as you choose Feelgood food, there is no counting Checks or measuring portions. For anything not Feelgood, count your Checks.

Portion control is still important. Even though you are not counting them, the calories are still there. Use the Eatwell Guide to see how much of each food group you should eat for healthy, balanced eating. Focus on consuming lean meat, vegetables, fruit and pulses whilst limiting your intake of high calorie, high fat and high sugar products.

IF YOU WERE MOSTLY B, TRY FOLLOWING CLASSIC CHECKS:

Maximum flexibility to eat the food you like, when you like. Every item of food and drink has a Check value attached. Simply count your Checks to stay within your daily or weekly allowance.

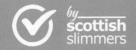

SETTING YOUR TARGET WEIGHT

When you are over-weight, losing any amount of weight will have a benefit for your health; research consistently shows that reducing your weight by 10% results in lowered blood pressure and reduced risk of developing Type II diabetes.

To achieve long term, sustainable weight-loss, we recommend a 5-10% weight loss goal - around 1kg or 2lbs each week - as a starting point.

Why? Simply, your Target Weight will be more sustainable with small steps, and with every goal reached providing the motivation to set and aim for the next one.

Remember, your Target Weight should be within the healthy BMI (Body Mass Index) range for your age and height. The Scottish Slimmers App will calculate and track this for you to stay within a range that's good for you.

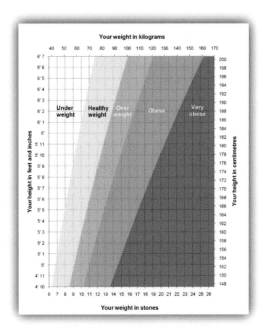

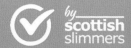

My 6 Week Milestones

Week	Weight	Waist
START		
WEEK 1		
WEEK 2		
WEEK 3		
WEEK 4		
WEEK 5		
WEEK 6		

WEIGHT LOSS:

Start ◯ Finish ◯ 6 week Loss ◯

CM / INCH LOSS

Start ◯ Finish ◯ 6 week Loss ◯

CLOTHES SIZE

Start ◯ Finish ◯

WHAT WILL YOU DO TO REACH YOUR TARGET IN THE NEXT 6 WEEKS?

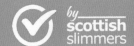

FEEL GOOD FOOD PLAN

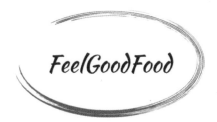

FeelGoodFood

What's great about Scottish Slimmers' FeelGood Food Plan is you can eat as much as you like. If this sounds too good to be true, read on.

Our FeelGood Food Plan encourages you to focus on the type of food you eat, to bring more balance to your eating habits and all to help you feel good, inside and out. Most of us don't eat enough fruit and vegetables, so we recommend they make up roughly half of your food intake on the FeelGood Food Plan.

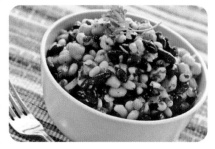

You'll find healthy, filling meals packed with fresh vegetables and fruits, dairy, eggs, high fibre pulses and wholegrains and pulses, plus lean meat and nutrient-packed fish. Stick to these and there's no need to weigh or count.

How does it work? Simply by cutting down, or cutting out, refined carbs, sugar and excess fat, you'll find your energy levels improve and, with more veg, pulses and protein, you'll feel full for longer. Use the app will manage your portion sizes, then you can eat what FeelGood Food you like, when you like.

Of course, Scottish Slimmers also believes nothing is off the menu, so you receive a FlexiCheck allowance each week to count any prepared, processed, or ready meals and treats.

FEELGOOD FOOD

FRUIT & VEGETABLES

Any fresh or frozen, or tinned in fruit juice.

Artichoke Apples Arugula Avocado Asparagus Bananas Beet Blackberries Broccoli Dates Brussel Sprouts Grapefruit Cabbage Grapes Carrots Kiwi Cauliflower Lemon Celery Lime Collard Greens Mango Cucumber Rhubarb Melon Endives Orange Fennel Peach Garlic Pear Kale Pineapple Leek Pomegranate Lettuce Strawberries Mushrooms Raspberries Squash Okra Onions Potato Spinach

PULSES, SEEDS & BEANS

Bean Sprouts Black Beans Black-Eyed Peas Chickpeas Green Beans Kidney Beans Lentils Mung Beans Peanuts Pinto Beans Soybeans Flax Hemp Pumpkin Quinoa Sesame Sunflower Chia Almonds Brazil Nuts Cashews Chestnuts Hazelnuts Pecans Pine Nuts Macadamias Pistachios Walnuts

LEAN MEAT

Any lean, trimmed, skinless meat.

Beef Chicken Duck Goose Rabbit Kidney Liver Mince* Pork Quail Pigeon Partridge Pheasant Rabbit Turkey Veal Venison

FISH

Any fresh or frozen (not coated with batter or breadcrumbs) or tinned in water or brine. Cod Haddock Salmon, Trout Sea Bass Herring Halibut Tuna Kippers Monkfish Perch Prawns Crab Shrimps Lobster Mussels Oysters Clams Cockles Whelks

any up to 10% fat

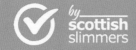

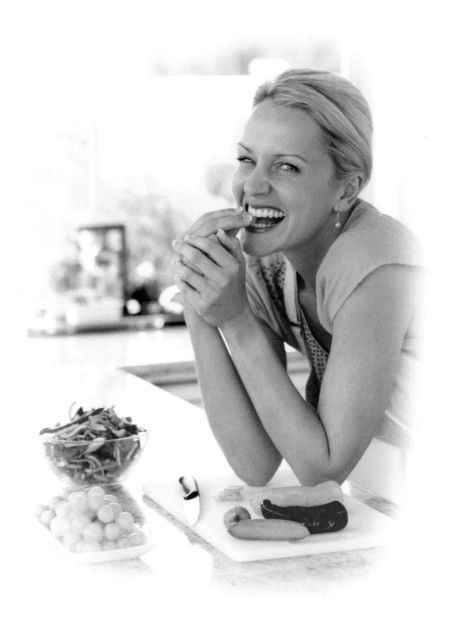

CLASSIC CHECKS PLAN

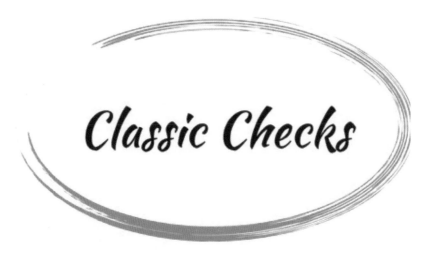

Scottish Slimmers' unique Check is our classic counting system, and it has been successful for more than 40 years, for tens of thousands of people just like you.

When life is full of choices, we make this one easy and with Classic Checks, you can achieve your best possible weight loss by tracking what you eat.

Our Classic Checks Eating Plan means that you can choose from thousands of foods, create your own meals and eat the food you love.

The Classic Checks Eating Plan has flexibility built-in so you can eat your favourite food when and how it suits you. You also have a weekly FlexiCheck allowance for the weekend, or to use for snacks or extra portions when you the mood takes you.

Every food and drink consumed has a Check value

100 calories = 4 Checks.

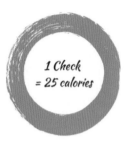

1 Check = 25 calories

With Classic Checks, there are only two important things to remember:

DAILY:

As you eat and drink, log in the App or count up the Checks you consume each and every day.

WEEKLY:

Use your FlexiChecks to top up daily or keep them for the weekends, special occasions or treats.

Simply by staying within your daily Check allowance, you will make great weight losses every week.

WEEKLY FLEXICHECKS

We help you make the lifestyle changes necessary to lose weight and, to get started, the amount of Checks you need each day in order to lose weight depends on your current body weight.

Look at your current weight range in the chart to find out how many daily Checks you need to eat to start losing weight. As you lose weight, your lighter body will require fewer calories, and Check allowances will reflect that.

Women			
Current Weight kg	Current Weight st lb	Daily Checks	Weekly Flexichecks
up to 65	up to 10.00	30	80
66 – 85	10.01 – 13.00	35	80
86 – 100	13.01 – 16.00	40	80
101 – 115	16.01 – 18.00	45	80
116 – 130	18.01 – 20.00	50	80
131 – 160	20.01 – 25.00	55	80
over 160	over 25.00	60	80
Men			
Current Weight kg	Current Weight st lb	Daily Checks	Weekly Flexichecks
up to 65	up to 10.00	50	120
66 – 85	10.01 – 13.00	55	120
86 – 100	13.01 – 16.00	60	120
101 – 115	16.01 – 18.00	65	120
116 – 130	18.01 – 20.00	70	120
131 – 160	20.01 – 25.00	75	120
over 160	over 25.00	80	120

Following Classic Checks will leave you feeling satisfied inside and out!

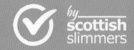

EVERYDAY ESSENTIALS

Some foods are more important to your health and well-being, they're essential to building balanced, nutritious eating habits, and should be included in your daily menus. We label these **Everyday Essentials**.

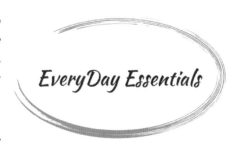

There are three categories of **Everyday Essentials**:

- ☑ *Fruit and veg for essential nutrients*
- ☑ *Good carbs for energy*
- ☑ *Dairy (calcium) for bone health*

*And the first **4 Checks** in each category are not counted towards your daily Checks allowance**

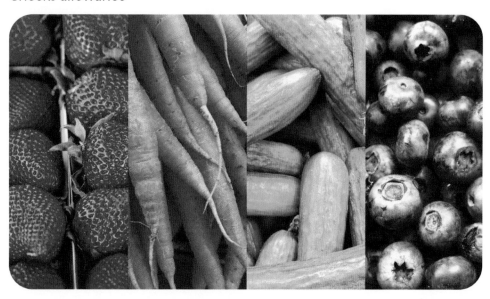

GOOD CARBS

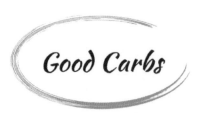

Confused about carbs? It's really no wonder. With headlines and articles giving the impression that "carbs are bad" many of us are confused about carbohydrates, although they play an important role for our health and to maintain a healthy weight. Even the word "carbohydrates" covers a wide category; not all carbs are equal so what's key is recognising the type, quality and quantity of carbs in our diet.

Starchy foods in themselves are not fattening, our bodies turn these starches, sugars and fibre into glucose, for the energy our bodies need to function. it's the added fats – eg butter or oil – frequently used in cooking or serving that increases the calorie content.

Scottish Slimmers recommends starchy foods such as brown rice, wholemeal pasta or cereals make up no more than one third of the food you eat, whichever Eating Plan you choose. On the app, Everyday Essentials badges help you keep track of your daily carbs*.

DON'T DITCH, SWITCH!

A small handful of plain, unsalted nuts – almonds, hazelnuts or peanuts - can have as much as 3g of fibre. Add raisins, sultanas or cranberries and you've a sweet snack any time of the day.

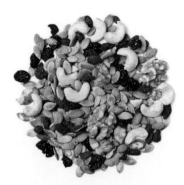

Buy brown rice or wholemeal pasta instead of processed white varieties.

Wholewheat or bread with grains or seeds, from your local baker, will have fewer additives and will be packed full of nutrients.

*Every day, the first 4 Good Carb Checks don't count for your daily Checks allowance**

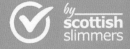

Consuming foods high in fibre gives that feeling of being full, contributes to a healthy digestive system and makes overeating less likely. You'll get most benefit from choosing wholegrain varieties, multi-grain bread and potatoes with their skins on, for their fibre content; **wheat, oats, barley, rye and rice** all come in wholegrain and provide slow-release energy.

TOP TEN TIPS

1. Replace cereals high in sugars for wholegrain cereals.

2. Plain porridge with fruit provides a filling, slow release of energy.

3. Overnight oats, easily prepared in jars or sealed containers to grab and go.

4. Adding raisins, nuts, bananas or strawberries to any cereal.

5. A baked potato for lunch, eating the skin for valuable fibre.

6. Cut the sauce and increase the veg with some brown rice or pasta.

7. Look for seeded, wholemeal and granary breads.

8. Versatile brown rice can make the basis of a tasty salad with and chopped veg.

9. Cauliflower rice is quick, delicious and with 15% of the Checks of traditional rice.

10. Complex carbs are full of nutrients as well as fibre found naturally in the food.

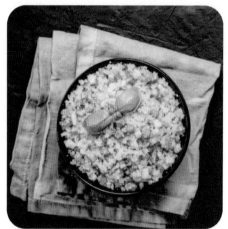

Evidence from nutritional research indicates that the fibre found in wholegrain starchy carbs is good for our health. Wholegrain cereals will contribute to your daily intake of iron, fibre, B vitamins and protein, and a diet rich in fibre is also associated with a lower risk of heart disease, stroke, type 2 diabetes and bowel cancer.

The Scottish Slimmers app recognises the first 4 Checks as No Check in your daily tracker.

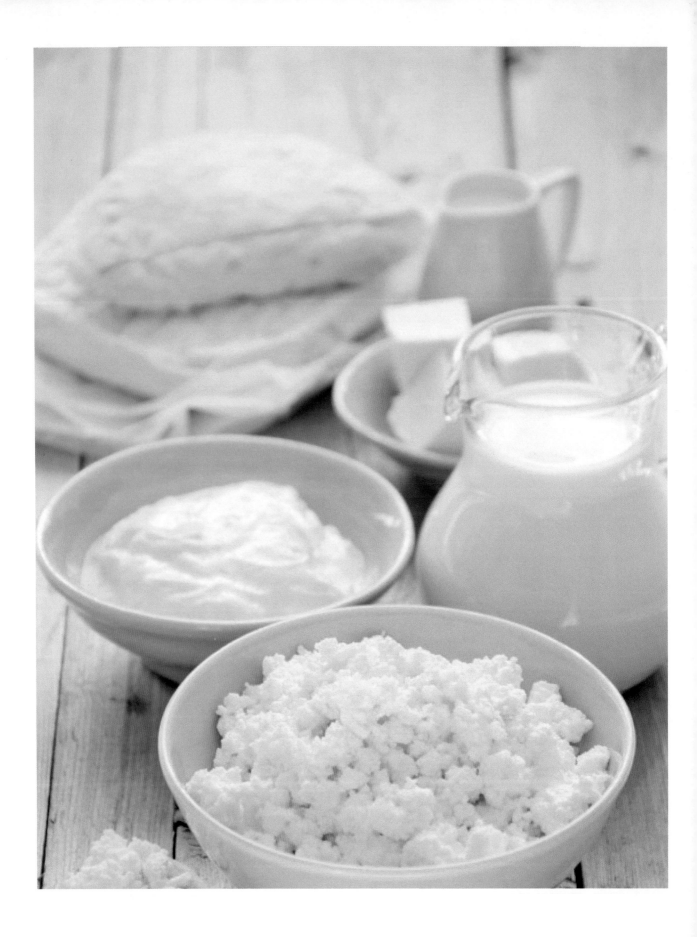

REMEMBER YOUR FLUIDS

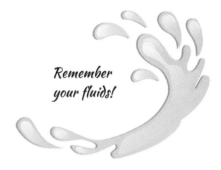

Remember your fluids!

At least 6 glasses of water every single day cost nothing, and can aid weight loss.

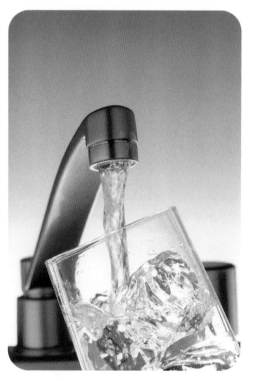

We don't recommend "diet" drinks, which are packed with artificial or processed sweeteners, so don't help build healthier habits.

If you really can't live without these, restrict them to one a day... we promise, you'll feel better for it.

FLEXI CHECKS

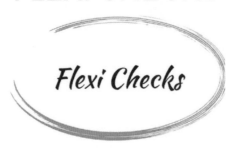

Both Eating Plans include the flexibility of FlexiChecks. Use your weekly FlexiChecks to top up your daily Checks on some days or to use when you have a special event or social 'eating and drinking' occasion to attend.

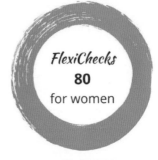

Women have 80 FlexiChecks, Men 120 FlexiChecks and it's up to you how you consume these. It might be a little extra each day during the week or spread over 2 or 3 days at the weekend. Whatever fits your lifestyle you have this allowance no matter which plan you follow.

With such a generous weekly FlexiCheck allowance there's no need to save daily Checks for the weekend.

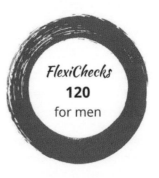

If you find you haven't quite used up all your Daily Checks in a day or your FlexiChecks within the week, it's best to forget them and start each week afresh.

Finally... Staying in Check

The important thing to remember is that counting Checks is simply a way of keeping the amount of food you eat under control – you don't need to be a wizard at counting, and you don't need to worry about the odd Check more or less, here or there.

GETTING STARTED

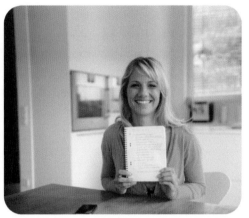

PLANNING...

We always recommend planning your meals and menus, then using this to create a shopping list

Red
eat occasionally

Amber
some of the time

Green
often as part of your diet

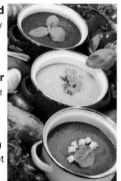

READ THE LABEL...

Food labelling breaks down the nutritional content of food, but are often full of information that can be difficult to understand, so we use these traffic lights for guidance.

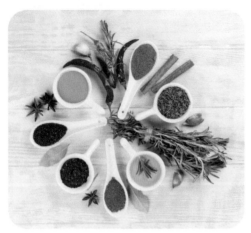

EAT WELL...

Search the Scottish Slimmers website or one of a dozen of our books for recipe inspiration nd menu suggestions. As you become familiar with Checks, you can be more creative

SIZE MATTERS

Check your portion sizes – a serving of meat should be roughly the size of your fist – and balance your meals so that you are heading for healthy not heavy. Vegetables should fill a third of your plate.

RED LIGHT

Red or processed meat can contain high levels of unhealthy saturated fat so try to reduce the amount you eat or avoid processed meat altogether. Always trim off any visible fat before cooking.

SWEET TREAT

A little bit of what you fancy is always good for your mood so enjoy your favourite sweet treat by all means but keep sugary foods to a minimum and as an occasional treat.

FISH FACTS

Oily fish such as salmon, sardines, mackerel and pilchards contain omega 3 essential fatty acids that are good for your heart and your brain. Aim to eat two portions of fish a week and make one of those an oily variety.

SNACK SMART

Swap sugary or high-fat snacks for something healthier like fruit or nuts. Picking these kinds of foods soon becomes a healthy habit.

JUST A PINCH

Salty food can slow down your weight losses, so reduce the amount of salt you eat by cutting back on what you add while cooking or at the table. Your taste buds will quickly adjust and any difference in taste will be temporary, but your body will thank you!

FILL UP WITH FIBRE

Foods high in fibre are fab, they fill you up, release their energy more slowly and keep you regular. Switch to wholegrain or wholemeal varieties and increase the amount of fruit, veg, pulses and grains you eat.

CHEERS!

From Prosecco to Pimms, you can spend your Checks on a glass of your favourite tipple* but choose wisely to get the best value from every Check. Generally, the more potent the drink, the higher the Checks.

Stay within your limit – health guidelines recommend no more than 2 units of alcohol a day on a regular basis. You should have some alcohol-free days every week.

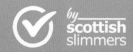

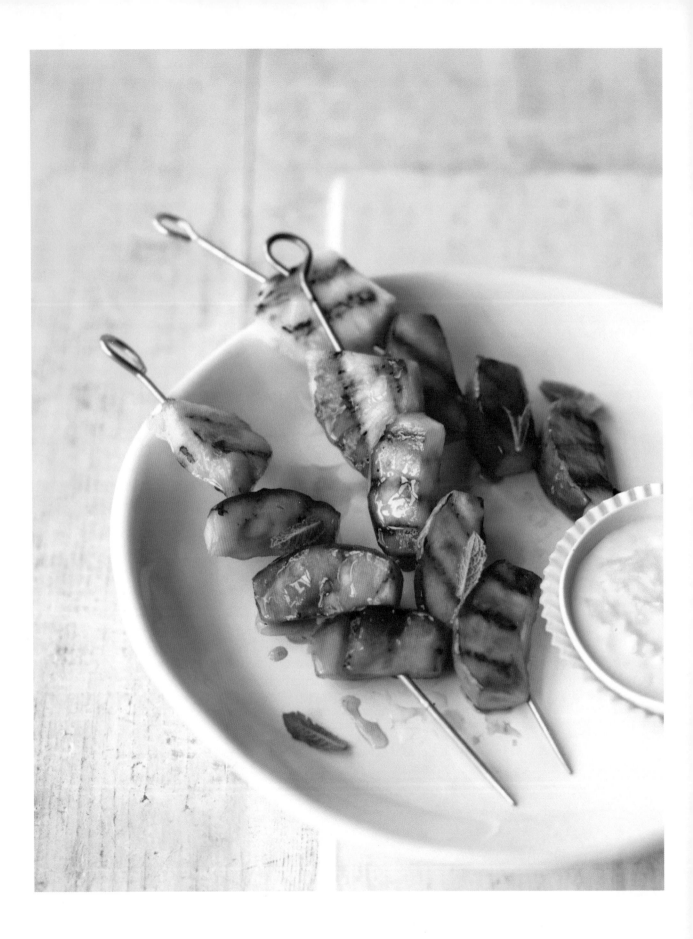

GET MOVING

"Is exercise important?"

A question frequently asked and can be answered, categorically – YES!

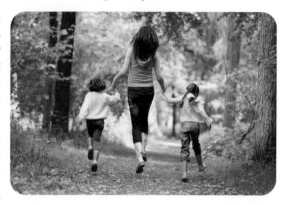

Exercise is a natural way to burn calories and, during your weight loss journey, will improve your body shape and muscle tone; it need not be vigorous just aim to be active in some way every day, and shopping, cooking or housework don't count!

Whether you love or loathe exercise, improving your physical fitness will improve your mental wellbeing too, it's one of the best ways to relieve stress or anxiety. Whatever your current activity level is, try to increase it. And, as a minimum, **aim for 30 mins every day**... your body – and the scales – will love you for it. Here's why:

HAPPINESS!

Getting your heart pumping relieves stress and can help alleviate depression by releasing endorphins – the 'happy hormones' that make you feel good about yourself

A SLIMMER FUTURE!

Burning calories and building lean muscle will help you lose weight and body fat – and inches -- as you tone up.

A HEALTHIER FUTURE.

Regular exercise reduces the risk of developing conditions such as type 2 diabetes, cancer and heart disease.

MORE ENERGY.

Whenever you start, better fitness will help you stay energetic as you age.

DEEPER SLEEP.

Being regularly active can lead to longer, better-quality sleep.

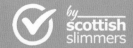

RECIPES

BREAKFASTS

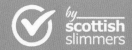

CHILLI VEGETABLE OMELETTE

SERVES 2 | 219 CALS PER SERVING | FG 2 | GC 0| CC 6

You'll need:

- 2 large eggs
- 50 g mangetout (shredded)
- 2 spring onions (shredded)
- ½ red pepper (deseeded and sliced)
- 1 tbsp Thai sweet chilli dipping sauce
- 1tbsp rice bran oil
- 2 tbsp fresh coriander (chopped)
- Salt and pepper to taste

Method:

1. Heat oil in a medium non-stick frying pan, add the vegetables and stir fry for 2 minutes.
2. Transfer to a dish and stir in the chilli sauce.
3. Beat the eggs in a bowl with coriander and seasoning.
4. Return the pan to a medium heat and pour in the beaten eggs.
5. Cook, stirring with a spatula to push the set egg to the centre of the pan, until there is no runny egg left.
6. Cook for a further 30 seconds until the base is golden.
7. Scatter the vegetables on top of the omelette and fold over.
8. Serve immediately.

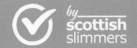

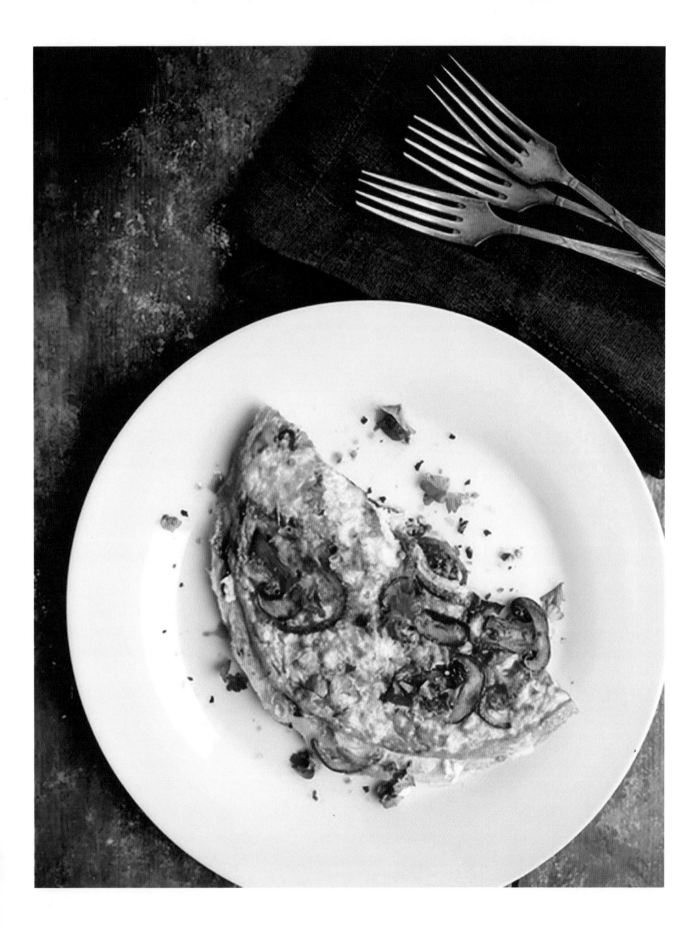

APPLE CINNAMON PORRIDGE

SERVES 2| 220 CALS PER SERVING | FG 0 | GC 1 | CC 7

You'll need:

- 60g porridge oats
- 180ml water or milk
- 1 red apple
- ½ tsp cinnamon

Method:

1. In a small saucepan, with your choice of water or milk, cook the porridge.

2. Grate the red apple, add to cooked porridge, and stir gently.

3. Sprinkle the cinnamon over and serve.

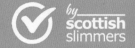

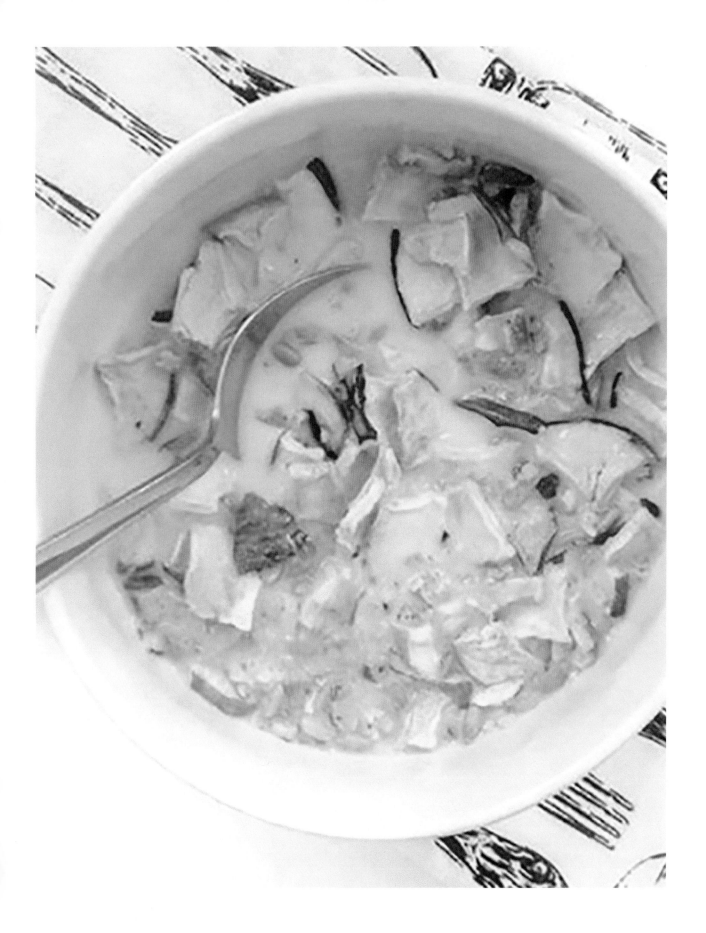

CREAMY MUSHROOMS ON TOAST:

SERVES 1 | 198 CALS PER SERVING| FG 0 | GC 1 | CC 8

You'll need:

- 2 slices wholemeal bread
- 25g low fat soft light cheese
- 100g chopped mushrooms
- ½ tsp mustard
- 1 tbsp chopped chives

Method:

1. Lightly toast the bread.
2. Mix the soft cheese, ½ tsp mustard and chives in a bowl.
3. Roughly chop the mushrooms and stir into the cheese.
4. Spread the mushroom mixture over the toast and heat under a grill for 3-4 mins.
5. Season to taste and serve.

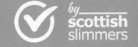

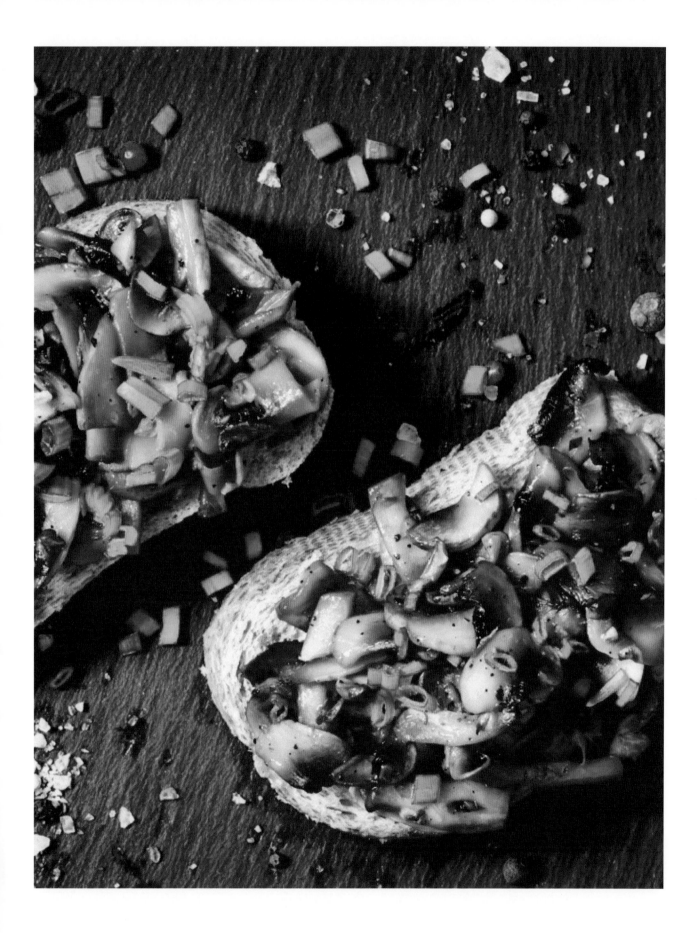

SMOKED SALMON BRUSCHETTA

SERVES 2 | 110 PER SERVE | FG 0 | CC 4

You'll need:

- 1 tsp horseradish
- 50 g extra light cheese
- 4 thin slices from a wholemeal baguette
- 120 g smoked salmon
- Chives or olives to serve.

Method:

1. Mix horseradish in a bowl with extra light cream cheese.
2. Season and mix well.
3. Lightly toast 4 thin slices from a whole meal baguette.
4. Spread the cream cheese mix over the toast, then layer the smoked salmon on top (approx. 30g per slice).
5. Add snipped chives or sliced olives to serve

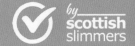

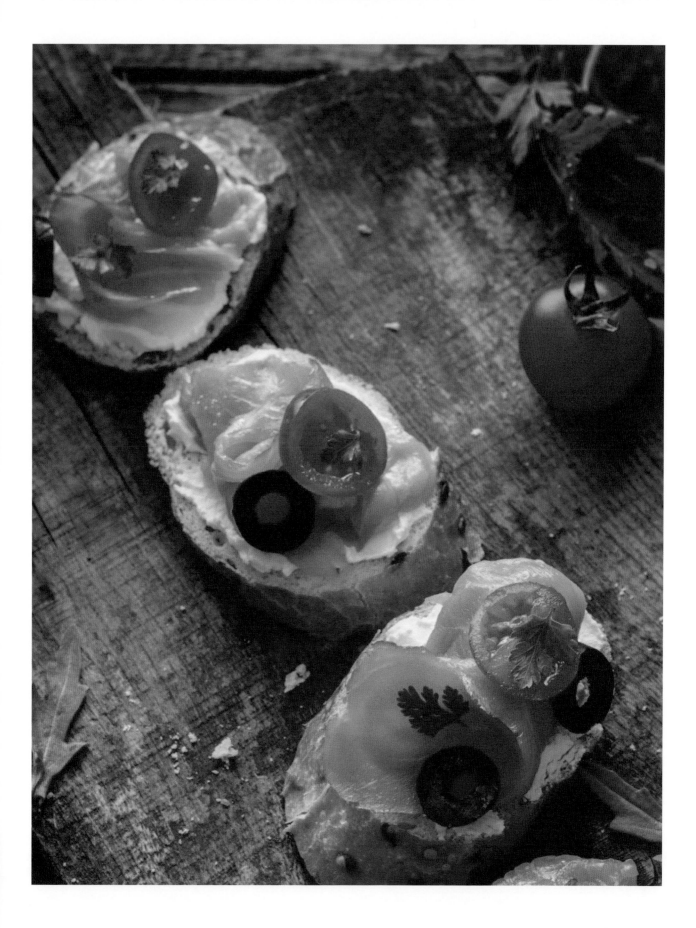

OVERNIGHT OATS

SERVES 4 | 286 CALS PER SERVING | FG 2 | GC 1 | CC 11

You'll need:

- 120 g porridge oats
- 100 ml unsweetened apple juice
- 200 ml water
- 2 apples- cored and grated
- grated zest of 1/2 orange
- 25 g walnuts
- 150 g 0% fat Greek yogurt
- 2 tsp clear honey
- 200 g berries
- 2 tsp sunflower seeds

Method:

1. Put oats, apple juice and water in a bowl. Cover and leave to soak overnight.
2. Before serving, stir in grated apple, orange zest, nuts and yogurt.
3. Divide between 4 serving bowls and drizzle with honey, berries and seeds.

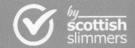

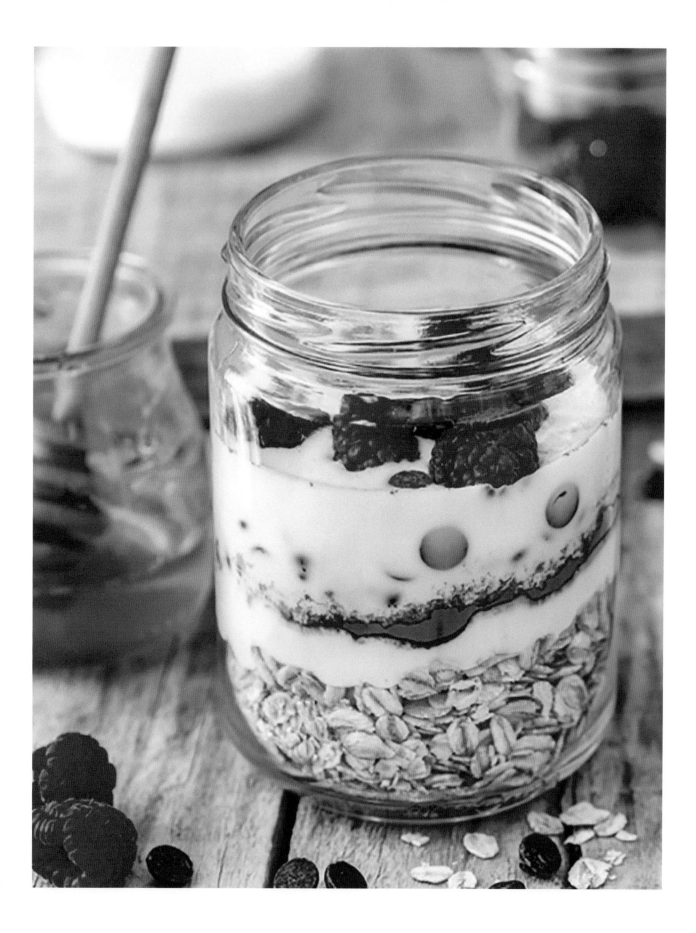

EASY EGGS FLORENTINE

SERVES 2 | 199 CALS PER SERVING | FG 0 | GC 1 | CC 8

You'll need:

- 2 large eggs
- 50g spinach
- 50g crème fraiche
- 2 tsp chopped dill
- 1 lemon
- 2 slices wholemeal bread

Method:

1. Wilt the spinach in a large pan with 50ml of hot water and juice of half lemon. Drain any water remaining and set aside.

2. Add the crème fraiche and chopped dill to the pan and warm over low heat, stir through half the spinach.

3. *Poach the eggs.

4. Toast the bread then add remaining spinach then spoon on fromage frais.

5. Top each slice of toast with a poached egg.

If poaching the eggs is a challenge, boil the eggs and cut in four to serve.

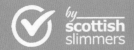

LUNCHES

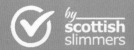

SWEETCORN AND COURGETTE FRITTERS

SERVES 4 | 163 CALS PER SERVING | FG 2 | GC 0 | CC 6

You'll need:

- 200g sweetcorn
- 2 spring onions
- 1 courgette
- 50g flour
- 1 egg
- 1 tsp mild chilli powder
- 2 tbsp milk
- 1 tbsp rice bran oil
- Handful spinach

Method:

1. Chop the spring onions, slice the courgettes, and mix with sweetcorn.
2. Beat the egg with dash of milk in a bowl then fold in flour and chilli powder to make a smooth, thick batter.
3. Stir in the vegetables to the batter mix.
4. Heat the oil in a large pan and spoon in 4 spoons of the mixture. Fry for approx. 3 minutes each side, which should be golden.
5. Season with salt and pepper then serve on a bed of spinach, or with steamed veg.

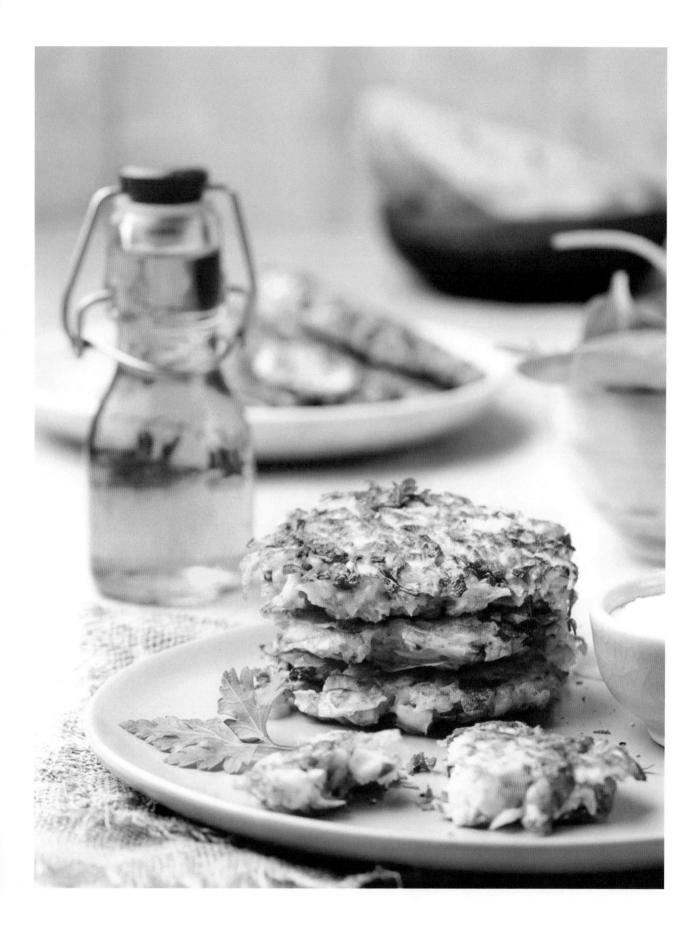

CHICKPEA WRAP

SERVES 2 | 422 CALORIES | FG 8 | GC 3 | CC 17

You'll need:

- 2 Wholemeal tortilla wraps
- 200g tinned chickpeas
- 1/2 avocado
- 1 stalk celery
- 40g red onions
- 2 tbsp light mayo
- Pinch of sea salt and ground pepper

Method:

1. Put the drained chickpeas into a big bowl with half the mayo and crush with a fork.
2. Add the avocado to the chickpeas and mash together.
3. Finely chop the celery and red onion, then add to the chickpeas and avocado.
4. Spread each tortilla wrap with the remaining mayo.
5. Divide the mixture into the wraps, and roll.
6. Serve with a green salad

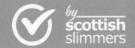

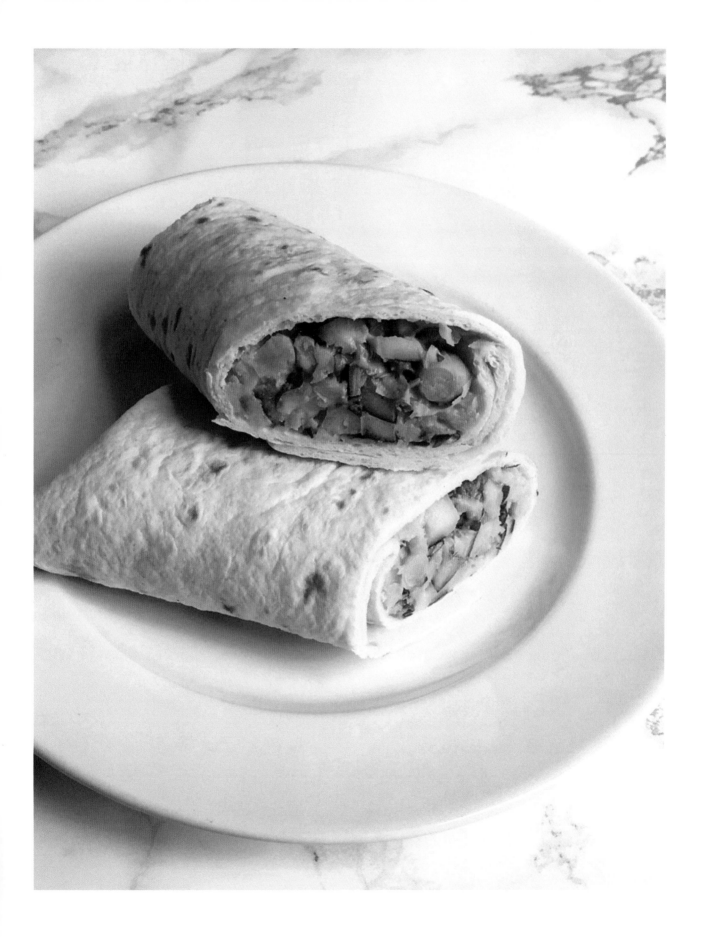

NOODLE JAR SALAD

SERVES 1 | 394 CALORIES | FG 9 | GC 3 | CC 16

You'll need:

For the dressing

- 1 tbsp peanut butter
- 2 tsp soy sauce
- 2 tsp Sesame oil
- ½ tsp chilli flakes
- 1 tsp rice wine vinegar
- Water

For the salad

- Large handful of frozen soya beans or tinned chickpeas (rinsed and drained)
- 100g fresh egg or udon noodles
- 1 stick of celery, sliced
- 4 radishes, sliced into wedges
- 1 spring onion, sliced
- 3 slices of Chinese leaf lettuce, finely shredded

Method:

1. Defrost the soya beans in boiling water then drain.

2. In a bowl whisk all the dressing ingredients with a splash of water until smooth. Pour into the bottom of the jar.

3. Layer the noodles on top of the dressing, then the celery and radish, then soya beans and

4. Top with the crunchy spring onions and Chinese leaf lettuce.

5. To serve, tip everything into a bowl and give a good stir.

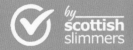

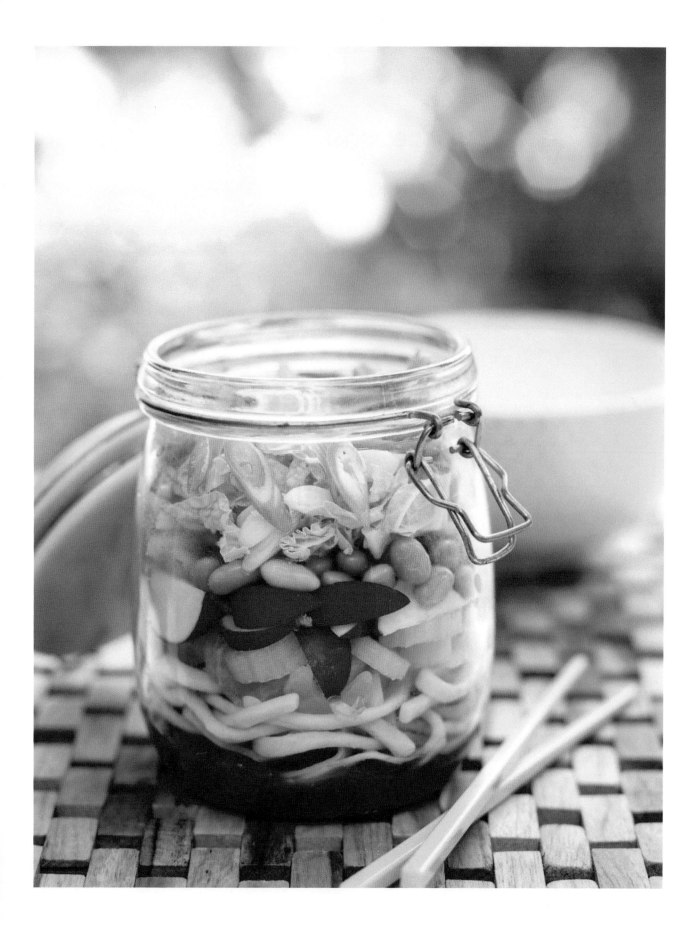

LOADED POTATO SKINS

SERVES 2| FG 0 | CC 7 | 181 CALS PER SERVING

You'll need:

- 2 Medium potatoes
- 1 Ripe tomato (chopped)
- 1 Spring onion (chopped)
- 30 g half-fat Cheddar cheese (grated)
- Salt and black pepper

Method:

1. Pre-heat the oven to 200 ˚C. Alternatively, cook in a microwave for approx. 8 minutes.

2. Scrub the potatoes and pierce them a couple of times with a skewer or fork before baking in the pre-heated oven for about 1 hour, until they are cooked and tender.

3. Halve the potatoes lengthways and scoop out most of the flesh (set this aside to use in another recipe).

4. Mix the chopped tomato and spring onion with the grated Cheddar cheese and a little seasoning.

5. Divide between the potato skins and pop under a pre-heated hot grill for about 3 minutes, until bubbling and golden brown.

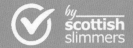

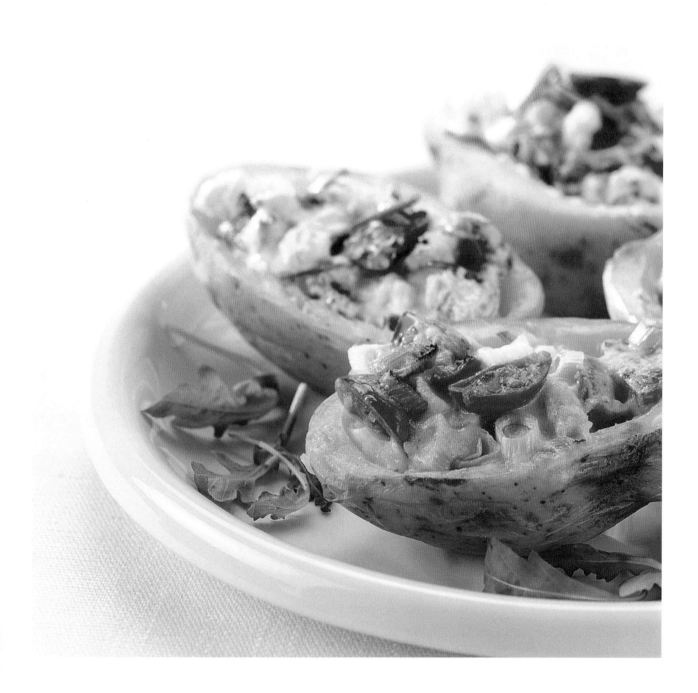

CARROT, CORIANDER & SWEET POTATO SOUP

SERVES 4 | 102 CALS PER SERVING | FG 0 | GC 1 | CC 4

You'll need:

- 500 ml chicken stock
- 3 carrots
- 1 large, sweet potato
- 2 leeks
- 200g chopped tomatoes
- 2 tsp Ground Coriander
- salt and pepper to taste

Method:

1. Chop up all your vegetables into chunks.
2. Slip the leeks and the carrots in a large pan.
3. Add the coriander and the chopped tomatoes.
4. Heat up the chicken stock (but do not boil) and then add it to the pan to to cover the vegetables by 1 - 2 inches.
5. Simmer until vegetables are soft.
6. Leave to cool. Once cooled blend until smooth or leave if you prefer chunky vegetables.

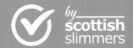

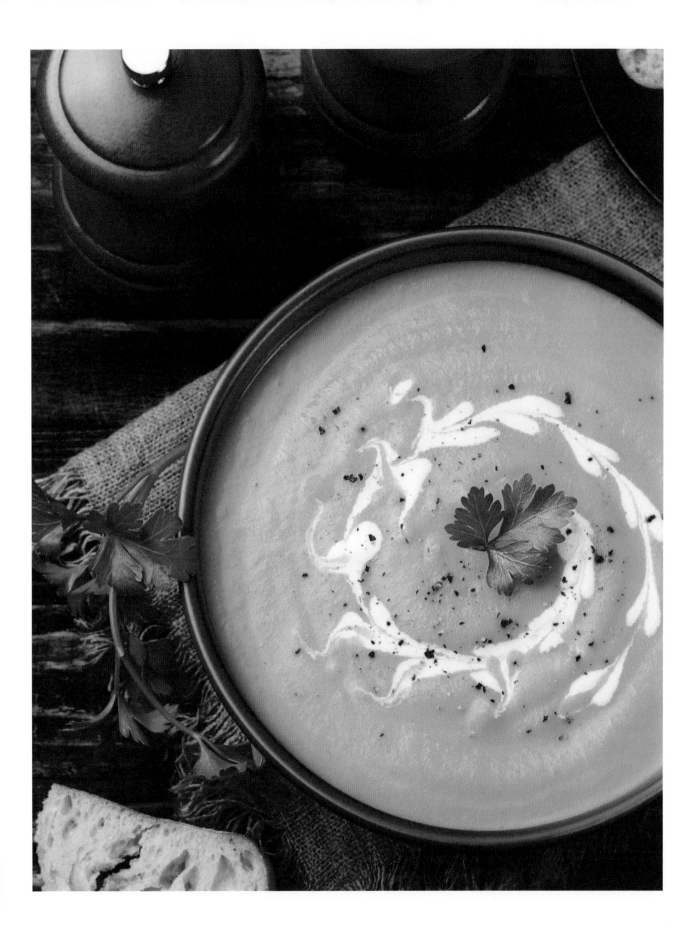

HAGGIS SOUP

SERVES 4 | 200 CALS SERVING | FG 4 | GC 0| CC 8

You'll need:

- 100 g Haggis
- 600 ml chicken stock (made with stock cube)
- 1 medium Leek (sliced)
- 1 small onion (chopped)
- 1 medium potato (peeled and diced)
- ½ small swede (peeled and diced)
- Salt and black pepper
- 1 tbsp rice bran, sunflower or similar.

Method:

1. In a stockpot, add the stock, potatoes and swede, bring to the boil and simmer for 15 minutes.

2. Heat the oil in a pan and cook leek and onion until soft.

3. Add the leek, onion and haggis to the stock, and simmer for 10 minutes, stir occasionally.

4. Season to taste.

5. Remove from the heat and spoon into bowls to serve.

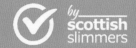

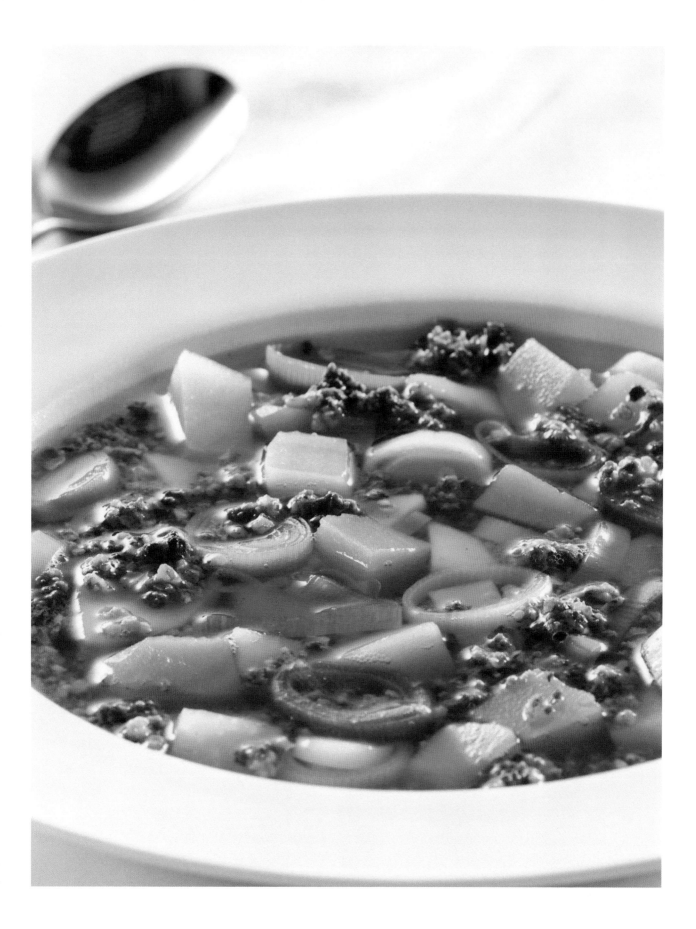

DINNERS

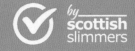

STILTON STUFFED CHICKEN BREAST

SERVES 4 | 268 CALS PER SERVING | FG 6 | GC 0| CC 11

You'll need:

- 4 chicken breasts
- 50g white Stilton
- 4 slices streaky bacon
- 12 cherry tomatoes

Method:

1. Preheat the oven 200c/400f gas mark.

2. Make a slit in the thickest part of the breasts with a sharp knife making sure not to cut through to the other side.

3. Divide the cheese into 4 and place in the pockets pulling the meat over to cover the cheese.

4. Stretch the bacon with the back of a knife. Wrap around each chicken breast making sure to cover the cheese.

5. Place in the oven and bake for about 20 - 22 minutes adding the cherry tomatoes after 12 minutes.

6. Serve with your choice of fresh or steamed vegetables.

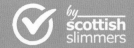

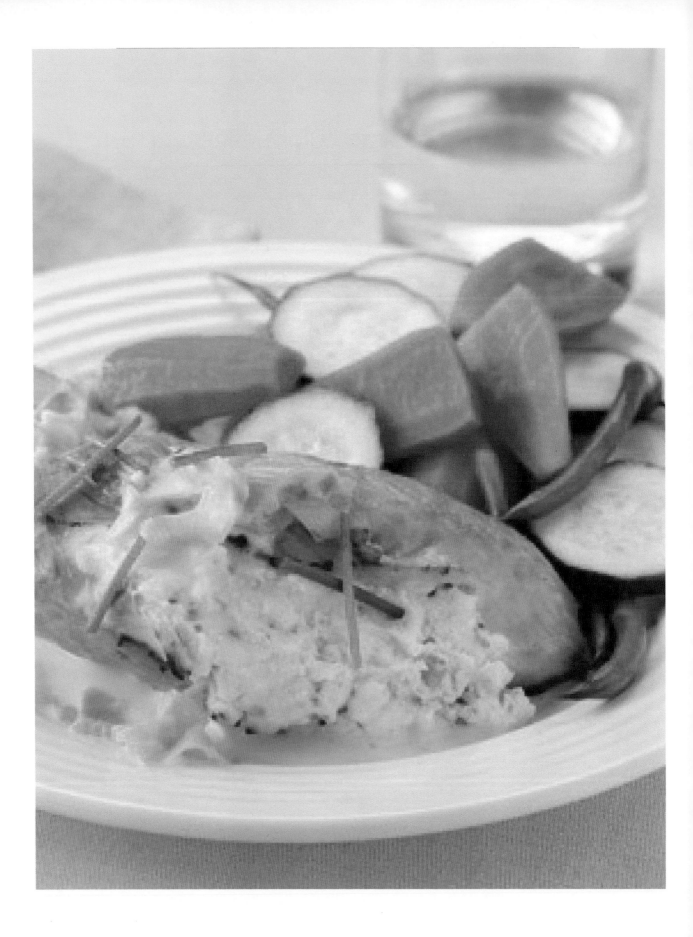

STUFFED AUBERGINE

SERVES 1 | 389 CALS PER SERVING | FG 0 | GC 0| CC 15

You'll need:

- 1 medium aubergine
- 1 onion (chopped)
- 1 medium carrot (diced)
- 1 medium stick celery (finely sliced)
- 1 tbsp tomato puree
- 8 cherry tomatoes (chopped)
- Pinch of mixed herbs
- Salt and pepper

Method:

1. Pre-heat oven to 200⁰C.

2. Cut aubergine in half lengthways. Scoop out and retain centres, leaving 2 shells. Sprinkle inside of shells with salt and pepper and place cut-side down on a baking tray. Bake for 20 minutes.

3. Put the onion, carrot, celery and chopped aubergine flesh into boiling water, then cover and cook gently for 10 minutes. Drain vegetables, crush or mash and stir in tomato puree, chopped tomatoes and herbs.

4. Remove shells from oven, turn over and fill with vegetable mixture. Return to oven for 10 minutes. Then serve.

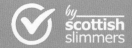

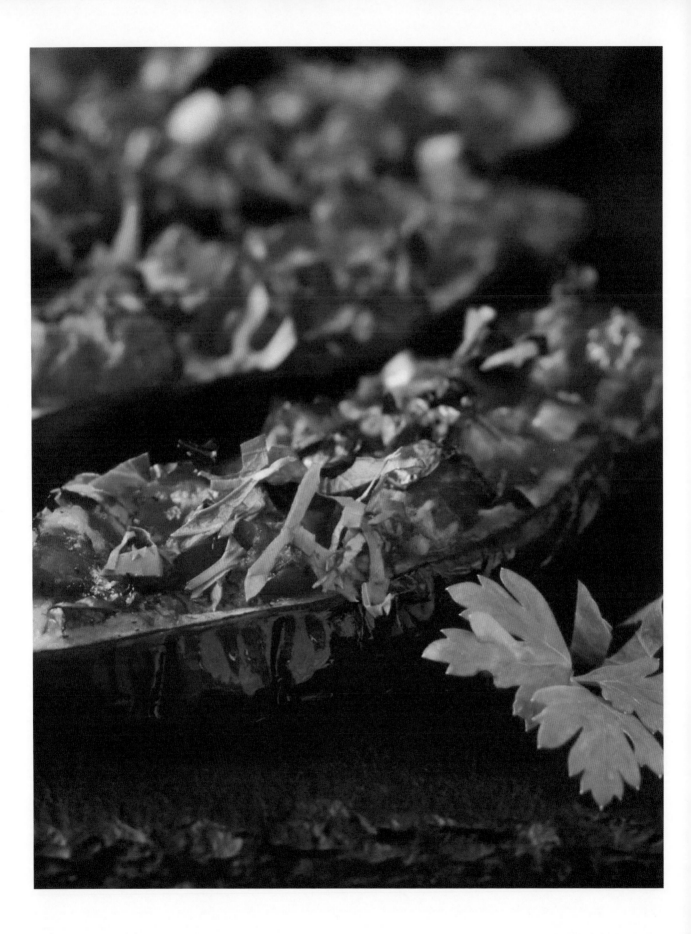

LEMON CHICKEN WITH BEANS

SERVES 4 | 225 CALS PER SERVING | FG 0 | CC 9

You'll need:

- 1 onion - chopped
- 4 x skinned chicken breasts
- 400g can cannellini beans, drained
- 500ml chicken stock
- Grated zest and juice of 1 lemon
- Few sprigs of oregano, tarragon or thyme
- Chopped parsley
- 1 tbsp rice bran oil

Method:

1. Spray a deep-frying pan lightly with oil and place over a low to medium heat. Cook the onion, stirring occasionally for 8-10 minutes until softened.

2. Add the chicken breasts and cook for about 6 minutes until browned on both sides.

3. Stir in the beans and then add chicken stock, lemon zest, juice and herbs. Turn up the heat and bring to the boil.

4. As soon as it starts to boil, reduce the heat and cook very gently for 15 minutes until chicken is cooked through and liquid has reduced and thickened a little. Add some ground black pepper.

5. Remove herb sprigs and serve, sprinkled with chopped parsley.

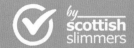

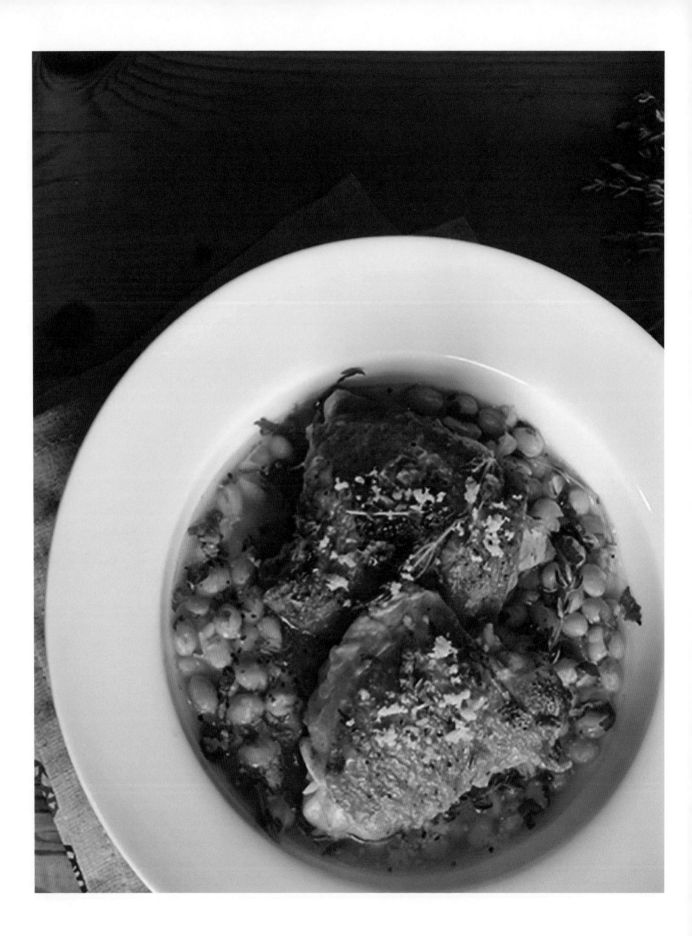

CHICKEN TIKKA MASALA

SERVES 2 | 326 CALS PER SERVING | FG 5 | GC 0 | CC 13

You'll need:

- 50 g Basmati rice (dry weight)
- 200 g Chopped skinless chicken breast fillets
- 200 g Canned chopped tomatoes
- 20 g Tikka Masala curry paste
- 100 g Red onions
- 1 clove Chopped garlic
- 1 tbsp rice bran oil

Method:

1. Cooked the basmati rice following the instructions on the package.
2. Heat the oil in a pan. Then, finely chop the onion and crush the garlic, add to the pan and cook until golden brown.
3. Add the chicken and cook through, add the curry paste to the garlic, onions and chicken.
4. Add the chopped tomatoes and simmer for 15 minutes until the chicken is tender.
5. Serve with cooked basmati rice.

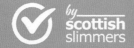

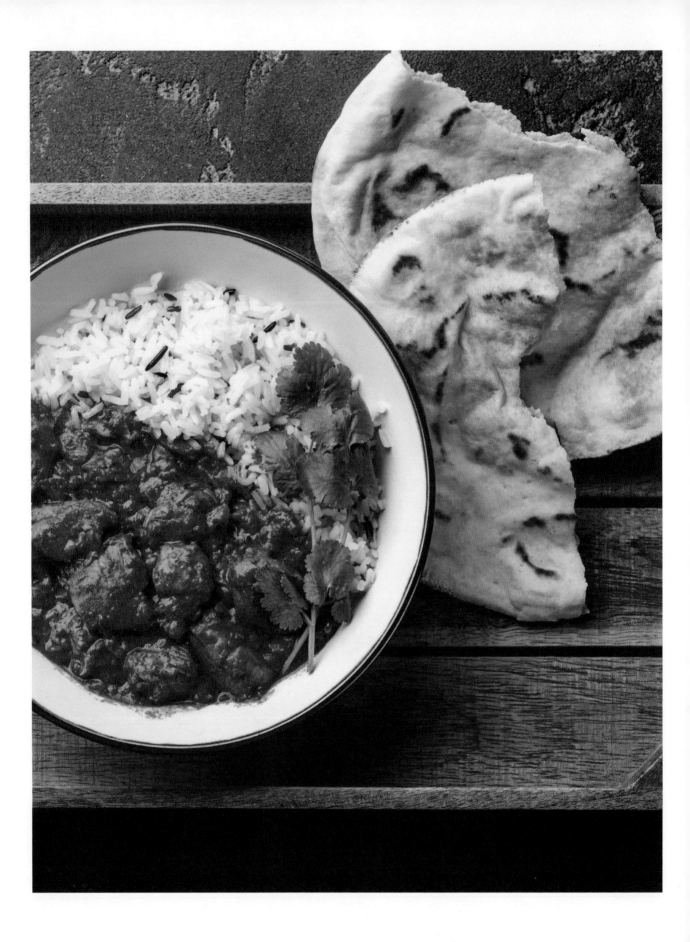

TURKEY BURGERS

SERVES 4 | 148 CALS PER SERVING | FG 1 | GC 0 | CC 6

You'll need:

- 400g lean turkey mince
- 1 red onion
- 100g dried apricots
- ½ tsp ginger
- Handful parsley
- 1 orange - zest and juice
- Olive oil

Method:

1. Mix turkey mince, grated red onion, diced apricots, grated ginger, chopped parsley, orange zest and juice in a bowl. Season with salt and pepper.

2. Divide mixture into 4 burger shapes. Cover and chill for 15 minutes.

3. Lightly spray the burger with oil and cook for 15 minutes until the juices run clear. Serve with salad.

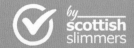

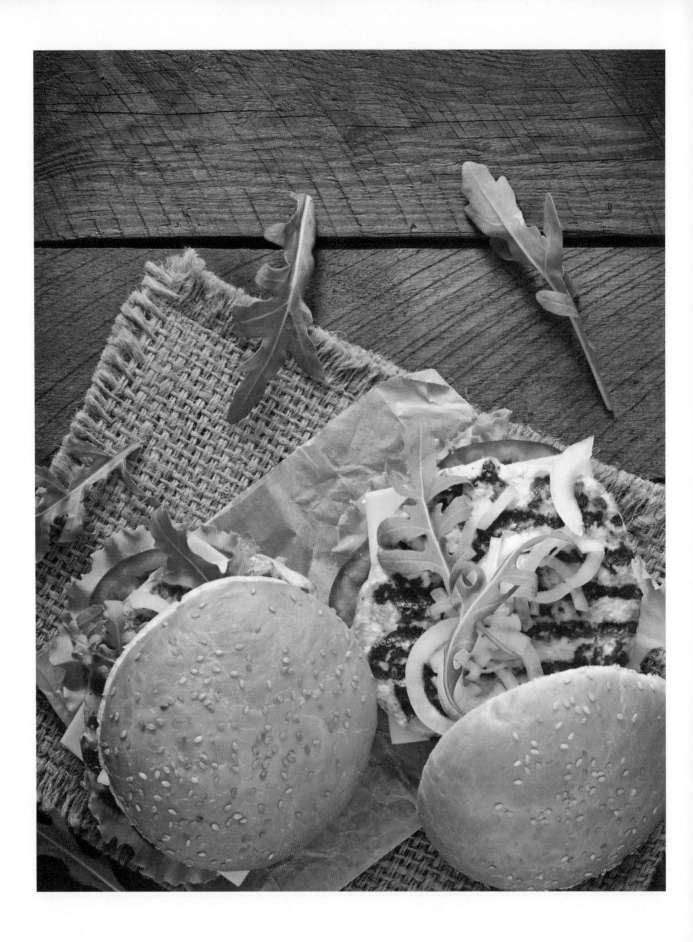

SWEET POTATO AND SPINACH CURRY

SERVES 4 | 280 CALS PER SERVING | FG 0 | GC 1 | CC 11

You'll need:

- 700g sweet potatoes (cut into chunks)
- 400g tinned chopped tomatoes
- 100g spinach
- 2 onions (thinly sliced)
- 2 tbsp curry powder*
- 1 tbsp rice bran or olive oil

Method:

1. Heat the oil in a large pot and soften the onions over medium heat.
2. Add curry powder and stir for 2 minutes.
3. Add potatoes, tomatoes plus 1 can of water, cover and simmer for 20 minutes.
4. Add spinach and cook until wilted.
5. Season and serve.

Alternative to premixed curry powder mix ½ tsp of each of chilli, coriander, cumin, fennel, fenugreek

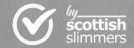

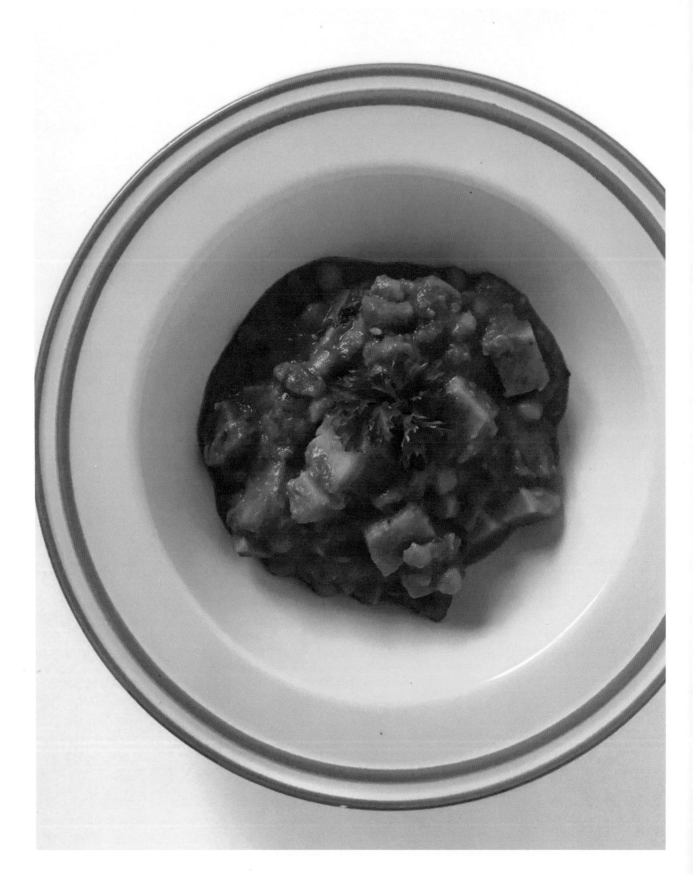

CHOCOLATE ORANGE POTS

SERVES 4 | 133 CALS PER SERVING | FG 4 | GC 0 | CC 6

You'll need:

- 60g dark chocolate
- 2 tsp cocoa powder
- 2 tablespoons hot water
- 2 eggs
- 1 tbsp caster sugar
- 1 tsp butter
- Grated zest of 1 orange
- Juice of ½ orange
- Peeled orange zest to decorate

Method:

1. Break the chocolate into pieces and place in a bowl over a saucepan of water. Mix the cocoa powder with hot water and add to melting chocolate. Stir until chocolate has melted and ingredients are combined, and mixture is thick. Remove from heat.

2. Separate the eggs into 2 bowls. Beat the yolks and stir into melted chocolate. Replace pan overheat and stir until sauce has thickened.

3. Add sugar, butter, orange zest and juice to melted chocolate.

4. Whisk egg whites until they form stiff peaks and fold gently into chocolate mixture.

5. Divide into 4 small dishes and chill in the fridge until set. Decorate with piece of orange peel.

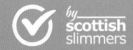

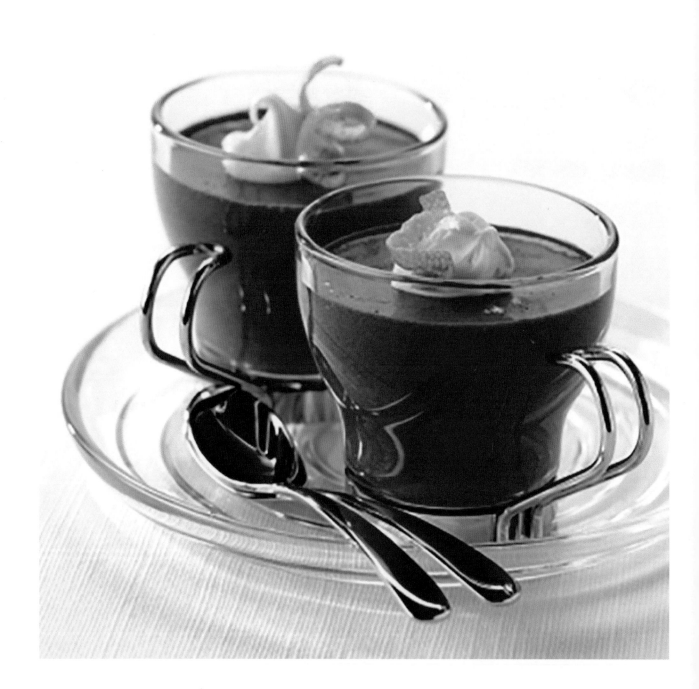

CHOCOLATE & RASPBERRY TRIFLE

SERVES 2 | 290 CALS PER SERVING | FG 8 | CC 11

You'll need:

- 1 chocolate-covered mini roll
- 2 tsp brandy
- 150 g frozen raspberries
- 150 g pot low fat custard
- ¼ tsp cocoa (optional)

Method:

1. Cut the mini roll into 6 slices and place 3 each in the bottom of 2 ramekins or glasses.

2. Reserve 6 raspberries for decoration and divide the remainder between the 2 dishes.

3. Sprinkle a teaspoon of brandy over the raspberries in each dish.

4. Divide the custard between the 2 dishes.

5. Put in the fridge for an hour or two so that the custard will seep through the raspberries as they defrost, and flavours will blend.

6. Just before serving, sift a little cocoa powder over the custard, if using, and garnish with the reserved raspberries.

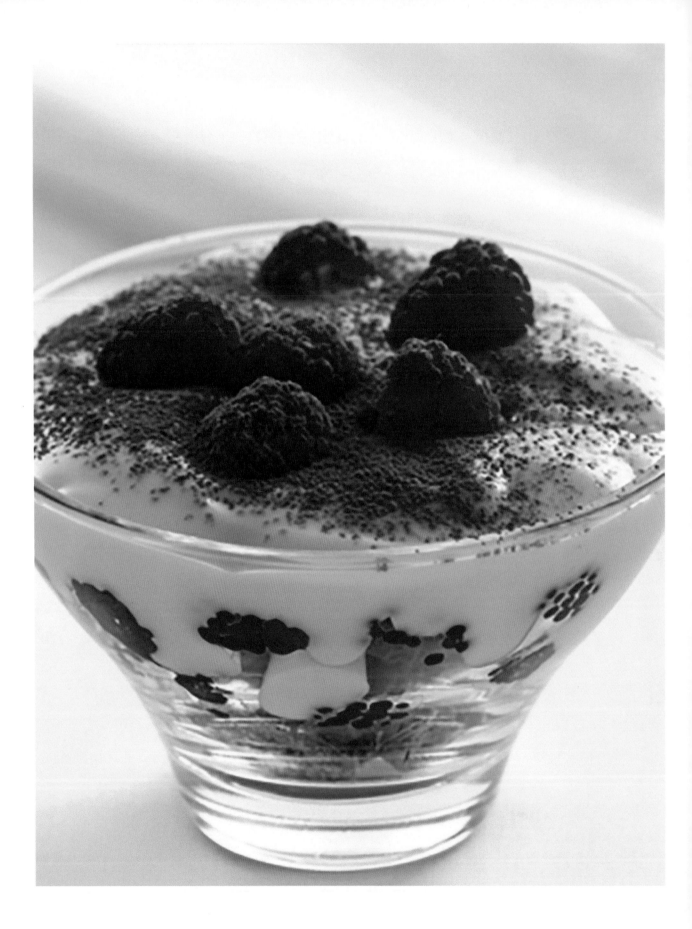

TIRAMISU:

SERVES 4 | 133 CALS PER SERVING | FG 2 | GC 0 | CC 6

You'll need:

- 8 sponge fingers
- 1 tbsp marsala
- 75ml cold black coffee
- 250g Quark or soft cheese
- 150g fat-free fromage frais
- ½ tsp vanilla essence
- 1 tbsp caster sugar
- Grating of dark chocolate

Method:

1. Break 8 sponge fingers into chunks and place in the bottom of 4 ramekins.
2. Stir vanilla and marsala into black coffee. Sprinkle coffee mixture over the sponge fingers.
3. Beat Quark and fromage frais until smooth then mix in sweetener to taste.
4. Divide mixture into 4 and spread over sponge fingers.
5. Grate over light covering of dark chocolate, cover and chill for 1 hour.

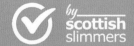

COCONUT CHIA PUDDING

SERVES 4 | 249 CALS PER SERVING | FG 4 | GC 0 | CC 6

You'll need:

- 1 Tin Coconut Milk
- 40 g Chia Seeds
- 1 Tbsp Maple Syrup
- 1 tsp Vanilla Extract
- 100 g Mixed Berries

Method:

1. Combine all of the ingredients in a bowl except the berries.
2. Stir well and then transfer the mixture to a sealed container.
3. Let the chia seed pudding sit in the refrigerator for 3 hours or overnight.
4. Once it is set, spoon into 4 bowls and serve with a handful of berries on top.

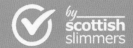

SPICED APPLE CRUMBLE

SERVES 6 | 206 CALS PER SERVING | FG 4 | GC 0| CC 8

You'll need:

- 450g cooking apples (peeled and cut into chunks)
- 1 tsp ground cinnamon
- 3 whole cloves
- Juice of ½ lemon
- 60g plain flour
- 60g rolled oats
- 30g low-fat spread
- 3 tbsp Demerara sugar

Method:

1. Pre-heat oven to 200°C/ gas mark 6.

2. Put the cooking apples in a saucepan with ½ tsp cinnamon, 1 tbsp of demerara sugar, whole cloves and lemon juice.

3. Cook gently over a low heat until the apples are slightly tender.

4. Sift the flour into a bowl and stir in oats and remaining cinnamon.

5. Gently rub in the low-fat spread with your fingertips until it resembles breadcrumbs. Stir in 1 tbsp sugar.

6. Put the apples into an ovenproof dish and cover with crumble mix, sprinkle over the remaining demerara sugar.

7. Bake in pre-heated oven for 25 minutes until golden and crisp.

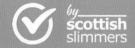

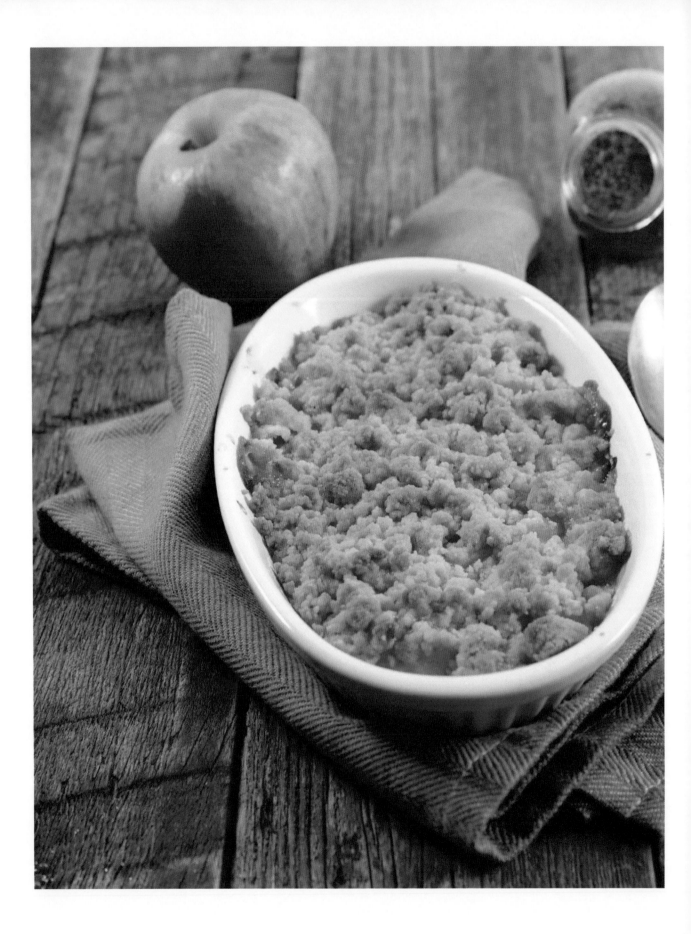

FEELGOOD FAIRY CAKES

SERVES 6 | 206 CALS PER SERVING | FG 2 | GC 0| CC 4

You'll need

- 4 separated eggs
- 250g quark
- ½ tbsp baking powder
- 5 tbsp granulated or half-spoon sugar
- 5 tbsp natural yogurt or fromage frais
- ½ tsp vanilla essence
- 6 strawberries
- 2 tbsp hot chocolate powder (optional)

Method

1. Separate your eggs, keeping whites in one dish and yolks in another. Using a whisk, beat the egg whites until thick.

2. 2 In the bowl with egg yolks, blend half (125g) of quark, baking powder, 4 tbsp sugar and vanilla essence. Once blended, whisk in half of the thickened egg whites.

3. 3 Then with a spoon, gently fold in the second half of the egg whites.

4. 4 Add mixture to 12 fairy cake cases. Bake in the oven at 180 degrees for 20 minutes. Allow to cool on a baking tray.

For the topping.

Mix the remainder of the quark with the fat-free natural yogurt and the remaining sugar

Spoon on to each cake, then top with chopped strawberries.

As an option, add 2 tbsp of hot chocolate powder for a delicious chocolate variation.

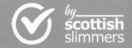

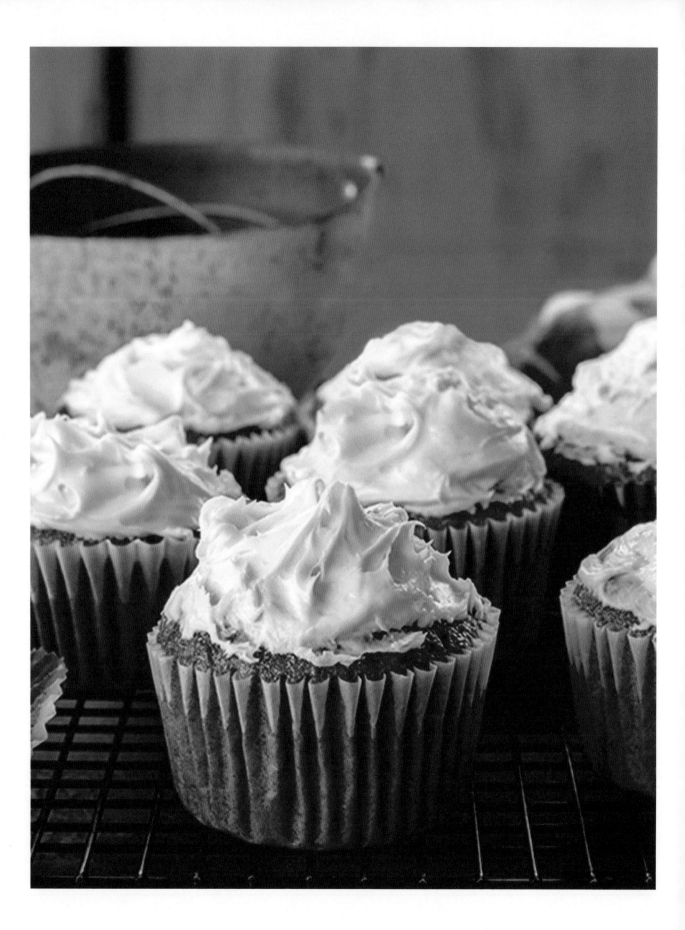

SNACKS & SWAPS

Don't ditch the dairy!

Numerous studies show calcium in the form of dairy foods, rather than supplements, appears to be far more effective at blasting belly fat.

SWAP semi-skimmed milk	FOR 1% fat or skimmed milk
SWAP full-fat Greek yogurt	FOR fat-free or 2% fat Greek yogurt
SWAP cheddar	FOR reduced-fat cheese, cottage cheese or quark
SWAP ice cream	FOR frozen low-fat yogurt

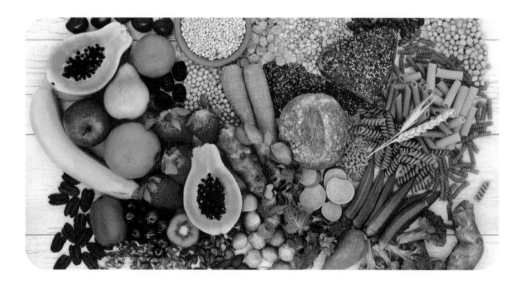

Shedding the processed carbs is a quick win. White bread, rice and pasta are easily swapped for much more nutritious wholegrains, such as wholewheat pasta, wholegrain cereals and breads, brown rice and oats.

SWAP cornflakes	FOR Shredded Wheat, Shreddies or Weetabix
SWAP white bread	FOR multigrain, rye or wholemeal bread
SWAP croissants	FOR wholemeal scones
SWAP white rice	FOR brown basmati rice

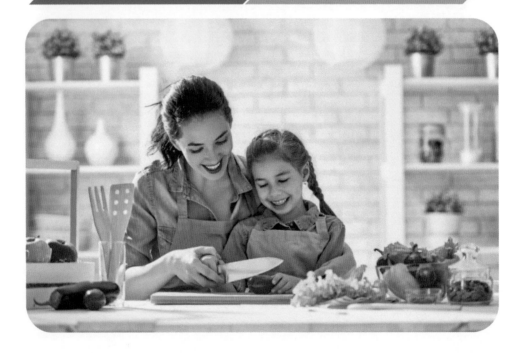

Not all fat is equal! Everyone should have a daily portion of heart-healthy monounsaturated fats – the kind found in olives and olive oil, avocados, nuts and seeds. Lean red meat and plain chocolate are also a good source. Just enjoy them in small amounts because all these foods have a high Check count.

SWAP butter	FOR peanut butter
SWAP sunflower oil	FOR rapeseed or olive oil
SWAP crisps	FOR a few unsalted nuts
SWAP mayonnaise	FOR olive-oil-based dressings
SWAP tortilla chips	FOR olives

GOT A QUESTION...

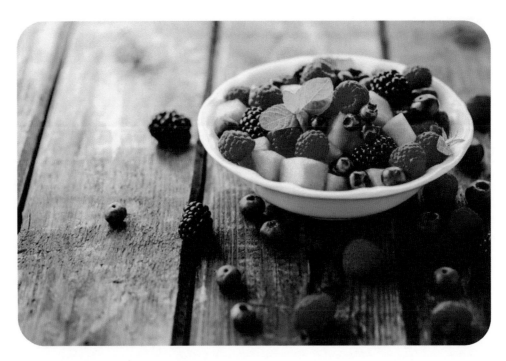

HOW MUCH CAN I LOSE?

Whether you follow Classic Checks or FeelGood, you can expect to lose around 1kg /2lb each week. Many people lose more in the first week or two, so don't worry if the losses reduce slightly after that time.

WHAT IF I WANT TO EAT SOMETHING THAT'S NOT INCLUDED ON THE FEELGOOD EATING PLAN?

Any foods not in the FeelGood categories have the same Check value as on the Classic Check system and these must be counted. After your EveryDay Essentials, your weekly FlexiChecks allowance should be used for these foods.

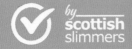

CAN I EAT FEELGOOD FOOD BETWEEN MEALS?

Yes, you can eat FeelGood Foods at any time. In fact, this plan is most effective if you have regular smaller meals or snacks to keep you going through throughout the day. We recommend keeping prepared vegetables or fruit handy, so your good habits aren't sabotaged by snack attacks!

WHAT IF I GO OVER MY WEEKLY CHECKS ALLOWANCE?

We all slip up sometimes, what's important is that you start every day with the intention to succeed. If it's just a Check or two, just cut back by the same number the next day. Or simply eat only food from the FeelGood categories for the next couple of days, remembering to count everything.

WHAT IF I DON'T USE ALL MY WEEKLY FLEXICHECKS ALLOWANCE?

Your allowances are designed to encourage healthy, sustainable eating habits. Provided you're using all your daily Checks, it doesn't matter if you don't use up every one of your weekly FlexiChecks BUT, never, ever "save" or carry over Checks.

WHAT IF I AM LOSING LESS THAN 1KG/ 2LB A WEEK?

Remember that everyone loses weight at a different rate. Lighter people, or those who are near Target Weight, will tend to lose at a slower rate than heavier people or those who have only recently started a weight loss plan.

If you're following the FeelGood plan, whilst you don't count FeelGood foods, perhaps you're eating too often, or the portions are too big?

Try this for one week: reduce your portions by 30-50% and only eat when you're hungry, this should reset your Plan.

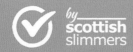

WHAT IF I WANT TO SWITCH BETWEEN FEELGOOD AND CLASSIC CHECKS?

Scottish Slimmers' Eating Plans are as much about creating sustainable habits, as losing weight, so we recommend you switch at the end of a week. This builds consistency and helps avoid mistakes ... or slip ups!

Remember, when you switch to the Classic Checks everything – apart from your EveryDay Essentials - has to be counted.

I HATE VEGETABLES, WHAT CAN I DO?

There are so many ways to cook or serve vegetables, it's unlikely you hate all of them! There are few foods that offer so much filling power for so few calories, and avoiding hunger pangs will help you stick to your plan. Vegetables also contain many nutrients that you simply can't get in sufficient amounts from other foods, so learn to love – at least some of - them.

WILL MY MEDICATION AFFECT MY WEIGHT LOSSES?

If you are prescribed medication, it's important to discuss any contraindications with your doctor or pharmacist. Following a balanced eating plan will help improve your long-term health, even if you are not losing weight quite as fast as you would like to.

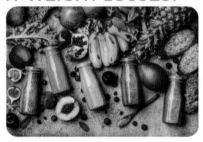

IF I EAT LESS, WILL IT SPEED UP MY WEIGHT LOSS?

Your Checks allowance is calculated to support healthy weight loss, which is sustainable over the long term, so it is really not a good idea to cut the recommend on a regular basis.

If you eat too little on a regular basis, your body response is to become more efficient at with fewer calories, making it extremely difficult to continue losing weight.

I HATE VEGETABLES, WHAT CAN I DO?

Different cooking methods bring out different flavours, so try stir-frying, roasting or steaming your veg, all much tastier than traditional boiling. And there are always creative ways to disguise or hide veg, grated into soups, casseroles or one-pot recipes, blended into sauces, dips or smoothies, it's endless, healthy and guilt-free!

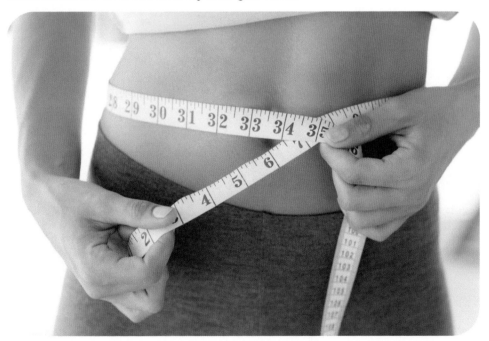

WILLPOWER AND WOBBLES

Let's face it, if this was effortless, we all be perfect!

Making healthier choices, whether that's eating more fruit and less fast food, or getting more active, on the days when we wobble, an element of willpower is essential to keep on track.

If you feel your self-control lacking – you're not the only one – here are the most common wobbles we hear, with our tips to avoid unhealthy habits creeping back.

I really deserved a loss this week and I've stayed the same. I'm so disappointed.

Sometimes weight can take time to shift. Measure your success in other ways. Take a couple of selfies every week, or take your body measurements, and compare each month, then you'll see the difference in how you look. Have a little patience, be kind to yourself and don't give up. Feel proud of your efforts and you'll get what you deserve in the end.

I want to feel good and look better but it seems like a long way off

If you're choosing from a menu in winter, it's hard to motivate yourself thinking about looking good on your summer holiday which is months away. It's easy to reward every step along the way – from the smallest a star in your diary or to a new pair of shoes, you choose! Having something to look forward to can keep you motivated. Break it down, think about your week ahead, and focus on each of the next 7 days.

I'm getting a bit bored with the meals I'm making.

Did you know that if you have as few as 30 breakfasts, 30 lunches and 30 main meals you have an astonishing 27,000 different daily menu combinations? Go to the Scottish Slimmers website for these, and more, meal ideas and build on your choice of recipes with some great Scottish Slimmers recipe books.

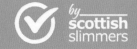

PLANNING TO SUCCEED

SUCCESS BINGO!

They say it takes 30 days to create or change habits, so set yourself up for success and aim to adopt at least one of these good habits every week for six weeks. By then, you'll see and feel the changes.

This is our version of success bingo, tick off each one as you do them and, by week six, you'll be well on your way to life-changing healthy habits.

1	2	3	4	5	6

1. Plan your meals, buying only the groceries on your list – and ignoring the cunning offers to fill your trolley!

2. Make cheating an effort by using an out of reach shelf or cupboard to keep tempting food out of sight.

3. Keep your hands and your mind busy – make a list of jobs you've been meaning to do, and do them!

4. Lace up your trainers and get outside EVERY day – aim to walk for at least 30 minutes, building up to an hour.

5. Weigh in once each week, and plan it. If you want to see real progress, hide the bathroom scales in between.

6. Write messages to yourself and stick them on doors and mirrors around the house as a reminder of why you're doing this.

Remember, when you think you've gone off track, simply enter everything you've eaten into your tracker, then close the day and start tomorrow with stronger resolve.

MEAL PLANNERS AND SHOPPING LISTS

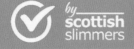

WEEK 1 MEAL PANNER

	Breakfast	Lunch	Dinner	Snacks
Monday				
Tuesday				
Wednesday				
Thursday				
Friday				
Saturday				
Sunday				

WEEK 1 SHOPPING LIST

Fruits & Veggies

_____

_____

_____

_____

Meat & Fish

_____

_____

_____

_____

Bakery

_____

_____

Store Cupboard

_____

_____

_____

_____

Non Food

_____

_____

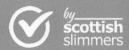

WEEK 2 MEAL PANNER

	Breakfast	Lunch	Dinner	Snacks
Monday				
Tuesday				
Wednesday				
Thursday				
Friday				
Saturday				
Sunday				

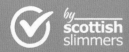

WEEK 2 SHOPPING LIST

Fruits & Veggies

_____

_____

_____

_____

Meat & Fish

_____

_____

_____

_____

Bakery

_____

_____

Store Cupboard

_____

_____

_____

_____

Non Food

_____

_____

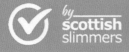

WEEK 3 MEAL PANNER

	Breakfast	Lunch	Dinner	Snacks
Monday				
Tuesday				
Wednesday				
Thursday				
Friday				
Saturday				
Sunday				

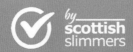

WEEK 3 SHOPPING LIST

Fruits & Veggies

_____

_____

_____

_____

Meat & Fish

_____

_____

_____

_____

Bakery

_____

_____

Store Cupboard

_____

_____

_____

_____

Non Food

_____

_____

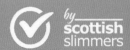

WEEK 4 MEAL PANNER

	Breakfast	Lunch	Dinner	Snacks
Monday				
Tuesday				
Wednesday				
Thursday				
Friday				
Saturday				
Sunday				

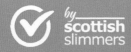

WEEK 4 SHOPPING LIST

Fruits & Veggies

_____

_____

_____

_____

Meat & Fish

_____

_____

_____

_____

Bakery

_____

_____

Store Cupboard

_____

_____

_____

_____

Non Food

_____

_____

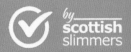

WEEK 5 MEAL PANNER

	Breakfast	Lunch	Dinner	Snacks
Monday				
Tuesday				
Wednesday				
Thursday				
Friday				
Saturday				
Sunday				

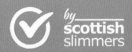

WEEK 5 SHOPPING LIST

Fruits & Veggies

_____

_____

_____

_____

Meat & Fish

_____

_____

_____

_____

Bakery

_____

_____

Store Cupboard

_____

_____

_____

_____

Non Food

_____

_____

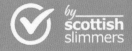

WEEK 6 MEAL PANNER

	Breakfast	Lunch	Dinner	Snacks
Monday				
Tuesday				
Wednesday				
Thursday				
Friday				
Saturday				
Sunday				

WEEK 6 SHOPPING LIST

Fruits & Veggies

_____

_____

_____

_____

Meat & Fish

_____

_____

_____

_____

Bakery

_____

_____

Store Cupboard

_____

_____

_____

_____

Non Food

_____

_____

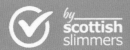

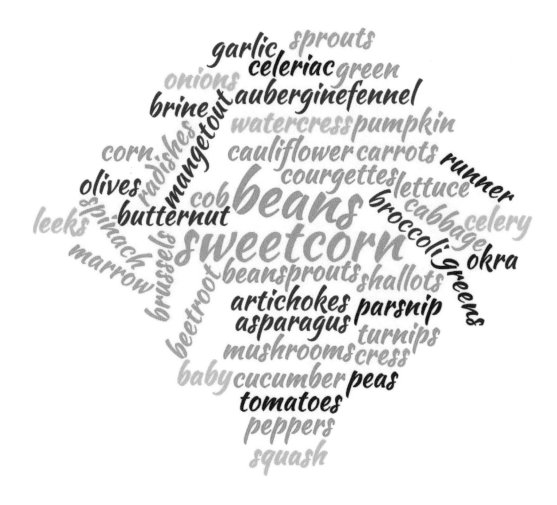

www.scottishslimmers.com

Printed in Great Britain
by Amazon